Paleo Smoothies

Refreshing and soothing paleo smoothies for those hot days!

Summary

- Easy/ understandable written structure

This book has been carefully designed to help the users and motivate them. In easily understandable English, this book is written to help a wide range of users of varying tastes. This book is designed to help readers save time. Because it is organized, the users do not have to read through irrelevant information before they find the smoothie recipe they are looking for.

- Easy Guideline

This book is published to educate and to motivate, and in order to do that a detailed table of content is given to help the users understand the structure of the book. Also the table of contents is linked to the smoothie recipes and you can easily jump onto the recipe of your choice by simply clicking on the link on the table of contents.

- Zero Redundancy

Only relevant information is used in the book. This book is especially designed to help customers and impart knowledge to them and not waste their time. Therefore, irrelevant or even extra information is avoided in this book, ingredients are listed down and right below that you will find specific instructions. The user is clearly able to find and act upon what they are looking for, which is what the target of the book is.

- Simple Ingredients

Most of the ingredients used in the recipes are simple and easily available. It has been made sure that extraordinary, difficult-to-find ingredients are avoided. In place of those, easy and readily available ingredients are substituted to enhance the cooking experience of the users. You will be able to experience great taste with simple ingredients.

- Numbered Steps for Recipes

Steps to accomplish the recipes are enumerated so the users find it easy to navigate through the recipe and prepare the recipes step wise and improve how you do things around the kitchen This way the users easily know which steps to complete first and which steps need completion. Dividing a recipe into milestones like this does not only make life easier, but also motivates.

Disclaimer and Terms of Use:

Effort has been made to ensure that the information in this book is accurate and complete, however, the author and the publisher do not warrant the accuracy of the information, text and graphics contained within the book due to the rapidly changing nature of science, research, known and unknown facts and internet. The Author and the publisher do not hold any responsibility for errors, omissions or contrary interpretation of the subject matter herein. This book is presented solely for motivational and informational purposes only.

Contents

Introduction

Another amazing e-book to help you in those hot days when the scorching heat calls for some chilled smoothies! Compiled with some amazing paleo smoothies to help you lose weight while enjoying food, this e-book has it all.

As you know, paleo makes use of a lot of fruits and vegetable and lean proteins to help you shed those extra pounds you have been working so hard to get rid off! With the use of some healthy fats, paleo diet is amazing!

People following the paleo diet have shown signs of improvement in health, such as improved lipids and reduced pain from autoimmunity, which other diets do not offer.

Moreover, people following the paleo diet have also shown signs of improvement in cardio vascular diseases. Research has shown that when compared to a Mediterranean diet, the paleo diet has scored more marks for the health benefits it brings.

Find some fine options in this book that will help you lose weight easily. Choose from the many recipes for smoothies and enjoy your hot summers!

Parsley Pear Green Smoothie

Serves One

Ingredients:

- 1 small bunch parsley

- ½ med avocados

- 6 med bananas

- 1 cup water

- 1 cup ice (200g)

- 1 nashi pear (aka Asian pear or apple pear)

- 1 pear

- 1 Royal Gala apple

- 1 Granny Smith apple

- 2 med plums

Instructions:

1. Peel and skin the avocados, banana, plums and apples. Remove any seeds.

2. Roughly chop the ingredients and put into a blender.

3. Blend until the smoothie is smooth and creamy.

Heart Healthy Reds

Serves One

Ingredients:

- 1 c. chopped red cabbage
- 1/2 red bell pepper

- 1/2 c. raspberries
- 8 oz. cold water
- 1 ice cube [optional]
- 1 tomato
- 5 medium strawberries

Instructions:

1. Roughly chop the ingredients and put into a blender with ice.

2. Blend until the smoothie is smooth and creamy.

Cherry and Kale Smoothie

Serves One

Ingredients:

- 1 cup of fresh or frozen cherries, remove pits

- 2 tbs. hemp seed

- 1 tbs. raw coconut oil

- 1 cup of ice

- 1 cup of fresh squeezed orange juice

- 1 cup of kale leaves, chopped

Instructions:

1. Roughly chop the ingredients and put into a blender with ice.

2. Blend until the smoothie is smooth and creamy.

Blueberry Avocado Power Smoothie

Serves One

Ingredients:

> 1 cup blueberries
>
> 1/2 ripe avocado, chopped-seed removed and peeled
>
> 1 tbsp coconut oil
>
> 1 apple, cored and diced
>
> 1 cup crushed ice
>
> 1 cup water or coconut milk
>
> 1/2 cup plain, full fat yoghurt
>
> 1 tbsp. almond butter

Instructions:

1. Take all the ingredients and put into a blender with ice.

2. Blend until the smoothie is smooth and creamy.

Peach Coconut Smoothie

Serves One

Ingredients:

1 cup full fat coconut milk, chilled

2 large fresh peaches, peeled and cut into chunks

fresh lemon zest, to taste

1 cup ice

Instructions:

1. Take all the ingredients and put into a blender with ice.

2. Blend until the smoothie is smooth and creamy.

Avacado Banana Smoothie

Serves One

Ingredients:

1 avocado, pitted

1/3 cup spinach

1/4-1/2 cup water

1 banana

Few cubes of ice

Instructions:

1. Roughly chop the ingredients and put into a blender with ice.

2. Blend until the smoothie is smooth and creamy.

Coconut-Cocoa-Macadamia Smoothie

Serves Two

Ingredients:

- 1 cup ice cubes

- 3/4 cup unsweetened coconut milk

- 2 tbsps. crushed salted macadamia nuts

- 2 tbsps. 'Swerve' or other sugar equivalent

- 1 tbsp. unsweetened cocoa powder

- 1/2 tsp vanilla extract

- 1 dash salt

Instructions:

1. Take all the ingredients and put into a blender with ice.

2. Blend until the smoothie is smooth and creamy.

Chocolate Bacon Smoothie

Serves One

Ingredients:

1 cup of coconut milk

1TB. of cocoa powder

1 banana

4 strips of cooked regular bacon (or 2 strips of thick bacon)

1TB. of honey or maple syrup

6-9 ice cubes

Instructions:

1. Take all the ingredients and put into a blender with ice.

2. Blend until the smoothie is smooth and creamy.

Green Spinach Smoothie with Apple

Serves Four

Ingredients:

- 1 Apple

- 1 Orange

- 1 C. Almond Milk

- 1 C. Ice Cubes

- 1/2 Lime – Peeled

- 1" Ginger (Frozen)

- 2 C. Spinach

Instructions:

1. Roughly chop the fruits and the spinach and put into a blender with ice.

2. Blend until the smoothie is smooth and creamy

Bulletproof Banana Smoothie

Serves One

Ingredients:

  1 cup Black coffee, chilled

  1/2 scoop Vanilla powder drink or PaleoMeal
  Vanilla Powder Drink

  1 tbsp. Almond butter

  1/4 cup Ice

  8-10 frozen banana chunks

  1-2 tbsp. Coconut butter

Instructions:

  1. Take all the ingredients and put into a blender with ice.

  2. Blend until the smoothie is smooth and creamy.

Creamy Pumpkin Cranberry Smoothie

Serves One

Ingredients:

1 cup preferred non-dairy milk

½ cup fresh pumpkin puree

¼ cup frozen fresh cranberries

2 tablespoons coconut cream (the fat atop a full-fat coconut milk can) or coconut butter

¾ teaspoon cinnamon

5-10 drops stevia liquid, to taste

¼ cup raw, soaked cashews

1 small apple, chunked

½ orange, peeled

Instructions:

1. Take all the ingredients and put into a blender.

2. Blend until the smoothie is smooth and creamy.

Banana Chai Smoothie

Serves One

Ingredients:

- 2 frozen bananas

- 2 tablespoons coconut milk

- 1/4 teaspoon each of vanilla, cinnamon, cloves and ginger

- 1 cup of water

Instructions:

1. Take all the ingredients and put into a blender.

2. Blend until the smoothie is smooth and creamy.

Creamy Orange Julius

Serves Three to Four

Ingredients:

 3 – 4 medium-sized oranges, peeled/de-veined/de-seeded

 1 can of coconut milk

 2 tbsps. honey

 Ice cubes

 1 tbsp. vanilla

Instructions:

1. Take all the ingredients and put into a blender.

2. Blend until the smoothie is smooth and creamy.

Paleo Strawberries and Cream Smoothie

Serves One

Ingredients:

- 1 cup frozen strawberries (not thawed)

- 1 tbs. raw cashews

- 1 tbs. raw honey

- 1 tbs. ground flax or hulled hemp hearts

- 1 medium ripe avocado, peeled, cored and diced

- 1 cup non-dairy milk or water

Instructions:

1. Take all the ingredients and put into a blender.

2. Blend until the smoothie is smooth and creamy.

Avacado Paleo Smoothie Recipe

Serves Three to Four

Ingredients:

1 avocado, peeled, cored and diced

2 frozen bananas, peeled and diced

1-2 tablespoons unsweetened cocoa powder

2 cups almond or coconut milk

½ cup frozen raspberries

Instructions:

1. Take all the ingredients and put into a blender.

2. Blend until the smoothie is smooth and creamy.

Warm Apple-Pie Smoothie

Serves One

Ingredients:

1 apple, cored and cut into chunks

½ cup / 120 ml water

¼ teaspoon vanilla extract

A pinch of nutmeg

A pinch of allspice

1 tablespoon maple syrup

¼ teaspoon ground cinnamon

1 scoop vanilla powder drink or PaleoMeal Vanilla Powder Drink (optional)

Instructions:

1. Take all the ingredients and put into a blender.

2. Blend until the smoothie is smooth and creamy.

Paleo Tropical Smoothie

Serves One

Ingredients:

1/4 pineapple, peeled and cubed

1 medium apple, cored and cubed

1 cup almond milk or coconut milk

1 banana, sliced

Instructions:

1. Take all the ingredients and put into a blender.

2. Blend until the smoothie is smooth and creamy.

Hunger Control Smoothie

Serves One

Ingredients:

1 banana, peeled and diced

1/2 avocado, peeled, seed removed and cubed

1c water

1 tbsp. true or Ceylon cinnamon

1-2 tbsp. coconut oil

1/4c coconut milk

Instructions:

1. Take all the ingredients and put into a blender.

2. Blend until the smoothie is smooth and creamy.

Sunshine Smoothie

Serves One

Ingredients:

Meat of 1 young Thai coconut

1 cup reserved coconut water

2 oranges, peeled

¼ tsp turmeric

1 cup ice

¼ cup beet kvass

2 bananas, peeled

2 TBS goji berries

¼ cup hemp seeds

Instructions:

1. Take all the ingredients and put into a blender.

2. Blend until the smoothie is smooth and creamy.

Sweetheart Smoothie

Serves Two

Ingredients:

1 Beet

One cup Kale

1 mango, peeled and diced

1 banana, peeled and diced

½ cup fresh pineapples

1 can coconut milk

2 tablespoons chia seeds

Instructions:

1. Take all the ingredients and put into a blender.

2. Blend until the smoothie is smooth and creamy.

Green Pina Colada Smoothie

Serves One

Ingredients:

1 cup coconut milk

2 tbsp organic shredded coconut (optional)

½ frozen banana

1 cup frozen pineapple chunks

1 cup spinach, packed

Instructions:

1. Take all the ingredients and put into a blender.

2. Blend until the smoothie is smooth and creamy.

Paleo Strawberry Clementine Smoothie

Serves One

Ingredients:

  2 clementine

  1 banana, frozen in chunks

  8 oz. strawberries, frozen

Instructions:

1. Take all the ingredients and put into a blender.

2. Blend until the smoothie is smooth and creamy.

Lean Green Smoothie

Serves One

Ingredients:

 2 oranges, peeled

 2 cups pineapple, chopped

 6 kale leaves, stalks removed

 2 cups mango kombucha

 2 cups water

Instructions:

 1. Take all the ingredients and put into a blender.

 2. Blend until the smoothie is smooth and creamy.

Guava Papaya Smoothie

Serves One

Ingredients:

> 1 cup ripe papaya, seeds removed, peeled and diced
>
> 2-3 Small guavas, seeds removed and chopped
>
> 1/2 Tsp ginger
>
> 1 Tsp maple syrup
>
> 1 sprig parsley
>
> 1 Tsp lemon juice
>
> 3-4 ice cubes

Instructions:

1. Take all the ingredients and put into a blender.

2. Blend until the smoothie is smooth and creamy.

Mango Almond Smoothie

Serves Two

Ingredients:

   3 ripe alphonso mangoes, peeled and chopped

   15-18 almonds

   sugar as required

   some ice cubes

   2-3 cardamom or ¼ tsp cardamom powder

   a few mint leaves for garnishing - optional

Instructions:

   1. Take all the ingredients and put into a blender.

   2. Blend until the smoothie is smooth and creamy.

Paleo Pumpkin Banana Smoothie

Serves One

Ingredients:

3/4 cups unsweetened almond milk

1 cup crushed ice

1/2 frozen banana

1/4 teaspoon each of cinnamon, nutmeg, and ginger

1 teaspoon finely ground flaxseed

1/3 cup pumpkin puree

1-1/2 tablespoons grade B maple syrup

Instructions:

1. Take all the ingredients and put into a blender.

2. Blend until the smoothie is smooth and creamy.

Chai Tea Smoothie

Serves One

Ingredients:

    1 cup milk of choice, warm

    1 chai tea bag

    ¼ tsp pure vanilla extract

    1 very-ripe frozen banana

Instructions:

1. In warm milk, dip tea bag and put into the fridge to let it chill. Throw away the teabag.

2. Take all the ingredients and put into a blender.

3. Blend until the smoothie is smooth and creamy.

Pink Monster Smoothie

Serves One

Ingredients:

One banana, peeled and diced

1 cup chopped pineapples

1 teaspoon honey

11/2 cup orange juice

21/2 cup red spinach leaves

Instructions:

1. Take all the ingredients and put into a blender.

2. Blend until the smoothie is smooth and creamy.

Mocha Chip Smoothie

Serves One

Ingredients:

- 1 cup brewed coffee (cold)
- 1 cup almond milk
- 1/2 banana (frozen)
- 1-2 medjool dates (pitted)
- 1 scoop of vanilla powder drink or PaleoMeal Vanilla Powder Drink
- 5-6 ice cubes
- 2-3 drops real vanilla extract
- 2 tsp cocoa powder
- 2 tbsp. hazelnuts or walnuts

Instructions:

1. Take all the ingredients and put into a blender.

2. Blend until the smoothie is smooth and creamy.

Cake Batter Smoothie

Serves One

Ingredients:

1 tablespoon macadamia nuts

1 tablespoon coconut butter

1 frozen banana

1 dried fig

1 scoop vanilla powder drink or PaleoMeal Vanilla Powder Drink

optional: honey and dark chocolate shavings to garnish

1 cup almond milk

½ teaspoon vanilla extract

¼ teaspoon almond extract

Instructions:

1. Take all the ingredients and put into a blender.

2. Blend until the smoothie is smooth and creamy.

Paleo Buttercup Smoothie

Serves Two to Three

Ingredients:

2-3 bananas, cut into 5 or 6 pieces each and frozen

1/2 cup almond butter

1-2 cups unsweetened coconut milk or almond milk

2-3 T cocoa powder

Instructions:

1. Take all the ingredients and put into a blender.

2. Blend until the smoothie is smooth and creamy.

Paleo Pumpkin Pie Smoothie

Serves One to Two

Ingredients:

1 frozen banana

2 tbsp. pumpkin puree

¼ tsp cinnamon

¼ tsp cloves

¼ tsp nutmeg

½ cup unsweetened almond milk

½ tsp vanilla extract

1 tsp honey

1 tbsp. hemp hearts

Instructions:

1. Take all the ingredients and put into a blender.

2. Blend until the smoothie is smooth and creamy.

Kale and Kiwi Smoothie

Serves One

Ingredients:

1 cup coconut water

1/3 cup ice cubes

1 kiwi, peeled and diced

1/2 pear

1 frozen banana

2 cups fresh kale leaves, stems removed

Instructions:

1. Take all the ingredients and put into a blender.

2. Blend until the smoothie is smooth and creamy.

Morning Paleo Smoothie

Serves One

Ingredients:

 1 can coconut milk

 1 cup frozen berries

 One raw egg yolk

 1 tbsp. nut butter

Instructions:

 1. Take all the ingredients and put into a blender.

 2. Blend until the smoothie is smooth and creamy.

Paleo Key Lime Smoothie

Serves One

Ingredients:

1 cup coconut milk

1 cup ice

honey, or sweetener of choice, to taste

½ avocado, peeled and diced with seed removed

zest and juice of 2 limes

Instructions:

1. Take all the ingredients and put into a blender.

2. Blend until the smoothie is smooth and creamy.

Expresso Protein Shake

Serves One

Ingredients:

½ cup cashew milk

½ banana, frozen

2 /3 cup ice cubes

¼ cup unflavored egg white protein powder

2 ounces espresso or strong coffee

½ teaspoon vanilla extract

dash of cinnamon

Instructions:

1. Take all the ingredients and put into a blender.

2. Blend until the smoothie is smooth and creamy.

Three Ingredient Smoothie

Serves One

Ingredients:

- 1 cup fresh baby spinach
- 1 cup frozen pineapple
- ¾ cup coconut milk

Instructions:

1. Take all the ingredients and put into a blender.

2. Blend until the smoothie is smooth and creamy.

Paleo Banana Bread Smoothie

Serves One

Ingredients:

1 cup cashew milk

2 frozen banana, sliced

fresh ground nutmeg, to taste

2 tablespoons almond butter

Instructions:

1. Take all the ingredients and put into a blender.

2. Blend until the smoothie is smooth and creamy.

Strawberry Coconut Smoothie

Serves One

Ingredients:

 1 cup coconut milk

 1 frozen banana, sliced

 1 teaspoon vanilla extract

 2 cups frozen strawberries

Instructions:

 1. Take all the ingredients and put into a blender.

 2. Blend until the smoothie is smooth and creamy.

Emerald Kale and Mango Smoothie

Serves Four

Ingredients:

1 mango, peeled, diced, stone removed

2 cups fresh kale – 2 large leaves, stem removed, leaves torn and washed

1 kiwifruit, peeled and diced

1 cup cold coconut milk

1/2 lime, juice only

Instructions:

1. Take all the ingredients and put into a blender.

2. Blend until the smoothie is smooth and creamy.

Salted Caramel Thick Shake

Serves One

Ingredients:

1/2 cup cold almond or coconut milk
1 1/2 tsp cashew butter/spread or 1/4 cup raw unsalted cashews, soaked

1/2 banana

2 dried pitted Medjool dates

1 tsp pure maple syrup

A pinch of sea salt

A couple of ice cubes

Instructions:

1. Take all the ingredients and put into a blender.

2. Blend until the smoothie is smooth and creamy.

Mixed Berry and Chocolate Paleo Smoothie

Serves One

Ingredients:

200-250ml coconut milk,

2 tbsp. PaleoMeal chocolate protein powder or paleo friendly chocolate powder drink

1 tsp of St. Dalfour Four Fruits fruit spread

Few cubes of ice

Instructions:

1. Take all the ingredients and put into a blender.

2. Blend until the smoothie is smooth and creamy.

Raspberry Mojito Smoothie

Serves One

Ingredients:

- 1 1/2 cup frozen raspberries

- 1 tsp coconut or maple syrup

- 1/2 cup orange juice

- 6-7 mint leaves

Instructions:

1. Take all the ingredients and put into a blender.

2. Blend until the smoothie is smooth and creamy.

Blueberry Acia Smoothie

Serves One

Ingredients:

1 cup coconut milk

1 1/2 frozen bananas

1 cup frozen strawberries

1 cup acai juice

1 cup frozen blueberries

3/4 cup ice

Instructions:

1. Take all the ingredients and put into a blender.

2. Blend until the smoothie is smooth and creamy.

Watermelon and Lime

Serves One

Ingredients:

3 cups chopped watermelon

1 lime, juice only

1 tsp honey or maple syrup

1 cup crushed ice or ice cubes

Instructions:

1. Take all the ingredients and put into a blender.

2. Blend until the smoothie is smooth and creamy.

Apple, Banana and Cinnamon Smoothie

Serves One

Ingredients:

- 1 cup chopped, peeled apples and diced

- 1 banana, peeled and diced

- 1 tsp cinnamon powder

- 1 cup coconut or almond milk

- 1/2 cup water

- 1 tsp vanilla essence/extract

- 1/4 cup unsalted almonds

Instructions:

1. Take all the ingredients and put into a blender.

2. Blend until the smoothie is smooth and creamy.

Blueberry Beetroot Smoothie

Serves one

Ingredients:

1 cup coconut milk

2/3 cup frozen blueberries

1 tbsp lime juice

1/2 cup ice cubes or crushed ice

1 medium beetroot, peeled and grated (including the juice)

Instructions:

1. Take all the ingredients and put into a blender.

2. Blend until the smoothie is smooth and creamy.

Toblerone Thickshake

Serves One

Ingredients:

4 dried dates

1/2 banana

1/3 cup hazelnuts

1 tsp honey

1 cup coconut or almond milk

A few ice cubes

1 tbsp cocoa powder

1/4 cup strong coffee

Instructions:

1. Take all the ingredients and put into a blender.

2. Blend until the smoothie is smooth and creamy.

Conclusion

Like you must have read, this book is especially designed for you so you can follow your paleo diet, enjoy the goodness of healthy fruits and vegetables and lose weight.

Similar recipes with simple ingredients incorporated simply in a blender, you will see how convenient and tasty these recipes are. We don't want your taste buds to die, so we have only provided recipes that will not only positively affect your health, it will also take your taste buds on a tasty joy ride of some fun smoothies.

Perfect for hot summer days, these paleo smoothies will rush through you and refresh your senses. Just take a few simple ingredients and toss them in a blender for a perfect smoothie!

Don't forget to enjoy your summers! Make some healthy paleo smoothies and give yourself and your loved ones a treat.

Good luck!

www.ingramcontent.com/pod-product-compliance
Lightning Source LLC
Chambersburg PA
CBHW070821290526
45795CB00002B/790